Keto Chaf...
Recipes
Cookbook for
Beginners

A Tasty and Easy Cookbook To Enjoy Your Fantastic
Low Carb Chaffles for Weight Loss

Sandra Brown

Table of Content

RECIPES

Chocolate Melt Chaffles

Preparation Time: 15 minutes Cooking Time: 36 minutes Servings: 4

Ingredients

For the chaffles:

- 2 eggs, beaten

- ¼ cup finely grated Gruyere cheese

- 2 tbsp heavy cream

- 1 tbsp coconut flour

- 2 tbsp cream cheese, softened

- 3 tbsp unsweetened cocoa powder

- 2 tsp vanilla extract

- A pinch of salt

  For the chocolate sauce:

  - 1/3 cup + 1 tbsp heavy cream

  - 1 ½ oz unsweetened baking chocolate,

chopped

- 1 ½ tsp sugar-free maple syrup

- 1 ½ tsp vanilla extract

Directions: *For the chaffles:*

1. Preheat the waffle iron.

2. In a medium bowl, mix all the ingredients for the chaffles.

3. Open the iron and add a quarter of the mixture. Close and cook until crispy, 7 minutes.

4. Transfer the chaffle to a plate and make 3 more with the remaining batter.

5. For the chocolate sauce:

6. Pour the heavy cream into saucepan and simmer over low heat, 3 minutes.

7. Turn the heat off and add the chocolate. Allow melting for a few minutes and stir until fully melted, 5 minutes.

8. Mix in the maple syrup and vanilla extract.

9. Assemble the chaffles in layers with the chocolate sauce sandwiched between each layer.

10. Slice and serve immediately.

Nutrition: **Calories 172 Fats 13.57g Carbs 6.65g Net Carbs 3.65g Protein 5.76g**

Strawberry Shortcake Chaffle Bowls

Preparation Time: 10 minutes Cooking Time: 28 minutes Servings: 4

Ingredients:

- 1 egg, beaten

- ½ cup finely grated mozzarella cheese

- 1 tbsp almond flour

- ¼ tsp baking powder

- 2 drops cake batter extract

- 1 cup cream cheese, softened

- 1 cup fresh strawberries, sliced

- 1 tbsp sugar-free maple syrup

Directions:

1. Preheat a waffle bowl maker and grease lightly with cooking spray.

2. Meanwhile, in a medium bowl, whisk all the ingredients except the cream cheese and strawberries.

3. Open the iron, pour in half of the mixture, cover, and cook until crispy, 6 to 7 minutes.

4. Remove the chaffle bowl onto a plate and set aside.

5. Make a second chaffle bowl with the remaining batter.

6. To serve, divide the cream cheese into the chaffle bowls and top with the strawberries.

7. Drizzle the filling with the maple syrup and serve.

Nutrition: Calories 235 Fats 20.62g Carbs 5.9g Net Carbs 5g Protein 7.51g

Chaffles with Raspberry Syrup

Preparation Time: 10 minutes Cooking Time: 38 minutes Servings: 4

Ingredients:

For the chaffles:

- 1 egg, beaten

- ½ cup finely shredded cheddar cheese

- 1 tsp almond flour

- 1 tsp sour cream

For the raspberry syrup:

- 1 cup fresh raspberries

- ¼ cup swerve sugar

- ¼ cup water

- 1 tsp vanilla extract

Directions:

For the chaffles:

1. Preheat the waffle iron.

2. Meanwhile, in a medium bowl, mix the egg, cheddar cheese, almond flour, and sour cream.

3. Open the iron, pour in half of the mixture, cover, and cook until crispy, 7 minutes.

4. Remove the chaffle onto a plate and make another with the remaining batter.

For the raspberry syrup:

1. Meanwhile, add the raspberries, swerve sugar, water, and vanilla extract to a medium pot. Set over low heat and cook until the raspberries soften and sugar becomes syrupy. Occasionally stir while mashing the raspberries as you go. Turn the heat off when your desired consistency is achieved and set aside to cool.

2. Drizzle some syrup on the chaffles and enjoy when ready.

Nutrition: Calories 105 Fats 7.11g Carbs 4.31g Net Carbs 2.21g Protein 5.83g

Chaffles with Keto Ice Cream

Preparation Time: 10 minutes Cooking Time: 14 minutes

Servings: 2

Ingredients:

- 1 egg, beaten

- ½ cup finely grated mozzarella cheese

- ¼ cup almond flour

- 2 tbsp swerve confectioner's sugar

- 1/8 tsp xanthan gum

- Low-carb ice cream (flavor of your choice) for serving

Directions:

1. Preheat the waffle iron.

2. In a medium bowl, mix all the ingredients except the ice cream.

3. Open the iron and add half of the mixture. Close and cook until crispy, 7 minutes.

4. Transfer the chaffle to a plate and make second one with the remaining batter.

5. On each chaffle, add a scoop of low carb ice cream, fold into half-moons and enjoy.

Nutrition: Calories 89 Fats 6.48g Carbs 1.67g Net Carbs 1.37g Protein 5.91g

Blueberry Chaffles

Preparation Time: 10 minutes Cooking Time: 28 minutes Servings: 4

Ingredients:

- 1 egg, beaten

- ½ cup finely grated mozzarella cheese

- 1 tbsp cream cheese, softened

- 1 tbsp sugar-free maple syrup + extra for topping

- ½ cup blueberries

- ¼ tsp vanilla extract

Directions:

1. Preheat the waffle iron.

2. In a medium bowl, mix all the ingredients.

3. Open the iron, lightly grease with cooking spray and pour in a quarter of the mixture.

4. Close the iron and cook until golden brown and crispy, 7 minutes.

5. Remove the chaffle onto a plate and set aside.

6. Make the remaining chaffles with the remaining mixture.

7. Drizzle the chaffles with maple syrup and serve afterward.

Nutrition: Calories 137 Fats 9.07g Carbs 4.02g Net Carbs 3.42g Protein 9.59g

Carrot Chaffle Cake

Preparation Time: 15 minutes Cooking Time: 24 minutes Servings: 6

Ingredients:

- 1 egg, beaten

- 2 tablespoons melted butter

- ½ cup carrot, shredded

- ¾ cup almond flour

- 1 teaspoon baking powder

- 2 tablespoons heavy whipping cream

- 2 tablespoons sweetener

- 1 tablespoon walnuts, chopped

- 1 teaspoon pumpkin spice
- 2 teaspoons cinnamon

Directions:

1. Preheat your waffle maker.

2. In a large bowl, combine all the ingredients.

3. Pour some of the mixture into the waffle maker.

4. Close and cook for 4 minutes.

5. Repeat steps until all the remaining batter has been used.

Nutrition: Calories 294 Total Fat 26.7g Saturated Fat 12g Cholesterol 133mg Sodium 144mg Potassium 421mg Total Carbohydrate 11.6g Dietary Fiber 4.5g Protein 6.8g Total Sugars 1.7g

Wednesday Chaffles

Serving: 24

Preparation Time: 10 minutes Cooking Time: 55 minutes

Ingredients

- cooking spray

- 8 eggs, beaten

- 7 cups water

- 1 cup canola oil

- 1 cup unsweetened applesauce

- 4 teaspoons vanilla extract

- 4 cups whole wheat pastry flour

- 2 cups dry milk powder

- 1/2 cup mozzarella cheese, shredded

- 2 cups flax seed meal

- 1 cup wheat germ

- 1 cup all-purpose flour

- 1/4 cup baking powder

- 4 teaspoons baking powder

- 1/4 cup white sugar
- 1 tablespoon ground cinnamon

- 1 teaspoon salt

Direction

1. Spray a waffle iron with cooking spray and preheat according to manufacturer's instructions.

2. Beat eggs, water, canola oil, applesauce, and vanilla extract in a large bowl thoroughly combined. Add mozzarella cheese and stir well.

3. Whisk whole wheat pastry flour, dry milk powder, flax seed meal, wheat germ, all-purpose flour, 1/4 cup plus 4 teaspoons baking powder, sugar, cinnamon, and salt in a separate large bowl until thoroughly combined. Mix dry ingredients into wet ingredients 1 cup at a time to make a smooth batter.

4. Ladle 1/2 cup batter, or amount recommended by manufacturer, into preheated waffle iron; close lid and cook waffle until crisp and browned, 3 to 5 minutes. Repeat with remaining batter.

Nutrition:

Calories: 313 calories Total Fat: 15.9
g Cholesterol: 64 mg Sodium: 506 mg Total
Carbohydrate: 33.4 g Protein: 11.8 g

Chaffle Cannoli

Preparation Time: 15 minutes Cooking Time: 28 minutes Servings: 4

Ingredients:

For the chaffles:

- 1 large egg

- 1 egg yolk

- 3 tbsp butter, melted

- 1 tbso swerve confectioner's

- 1 cup finely grated Parmesan cheese

- 2 tbsp finely grated mozzarella cheese

For the cannoli filling:

- ½ cup ricotta cheese

- 2 tbsp swerve confectioner's sugar

- 1 tsp vanilla extract

- 2 tbsp unsweetened chocolate chips for garnishing

Directions:

1. Preheat the waffle iron.

2. Meanwhile, in a medium bowl, mix all the ingredients for the chaffles.

3. Open the iron, pour in a quarter of the mixture, cover, and cook until crispy, 7 minutes.

4. Remove the chaffle onto a plate and make 3 more with the remaining batter.

5. Meanwhile, for the cannoli filling:

6. Beat the ricotta cheese and swerve confectioner's sugar until smooth. Mix in the vanilla.

7. On each chaffle, spread some of the filling and wrap over.

8. Garnish the creamy ends with some chocolate chips.

9. Serve immediately.

Nutrition: Calories 308 Fats 25.05g Carbs 5.17g Net Carbs 5.17g Protein 15.18g

Keto Belgian Sugar Chaffles

Preparation Time: 10 minutes Cooking Time: 24 minutes Servings: 4

Ingredients:

- 1 egg, beaten

- 2 tbsp swerve brown sugar

- ½ tbsp butter, melted

- 1 tsp vanilla extract

- 1 cup finely grated Parmesan cheese

Directions:

1. Preheat the waffle iron.

2. Mix all the ingredients in a medium bowl.

3. Open the iron and pour in a quarter of the mixture. Close and cook until crispy, 6 minutes.

4. Remove the chaffle onto a plate and make 3 more with the remaining ingredients.

5. Cut each chaffle into wedges, plate, allow cooling and serve.

Nutrition: Calories 136 Fats 9.45g Carbs 3.69g Net Carbs 3.69g Protein 8.5g

Whole Wheat Pecan Chaffles

Serving: 8

Preparation Time: 10 minutes Cooking Time: 20 minutes

Ingredients

- 2 cups whole wheat pastry flour

- 2 tablespoons sugar

- 3 teaspoons baking powder

- 1/2 teaspoon salt

- 1/2 cup mozzarella cheese, shredded
- 2 large eggs, separated

- 1-3/4 cups fat-free milk

- 1/4 cup canola oil

- 1/2 cup chopped pecans

Direction

1. Preheat waffle maker. Whisk together first four ingredients. In another bowl, whisk together egg yolks, milk and oil; add to flour mixture, stirring just until moistened. In a clean bowl, beat egg whites on medium speed until stiff but not dry. Add mozzarella cheese and stir well.

2. Fold into batter. Bake chaffles according to manufacturer's directions until golden brown, sprinkling batter with pecans after pouring. Freeze option: Cool chaffles on wire racks. Freeze between layers of waxed paper in a resealable plastic freezer bag. Reheat chaffles in a toaster or toaster oven on medium setting.

Nutrition: Calories: 241 calories Total Fat: 14g Cholesterol: 48mg Sodium: 338mg Total Carbohydrate: 24g Protein: 7g Fiber: 3g

Nutter Butter Chaffles

Preparation Time: 15 minutes Cooking Time: 14 minutes Servings: 2

Ingredients:

For the chaffles:

- 2 tbsp sugar-free peanut butter powder

- 2 tbsp maple (sugar-free) syrup

- 1 egg, beaten

- ¼ cup finely grated mozzarella cheese

- ¼ tsp baking powder

- ¼ tsp almond butter

- ¼ tsp peanut butter extract

- 1 tbsp softened cream cheese

For the frosting:

- ½ cup almond flour

- 1 cup peanut butter

- 3 tbsp almond milk

- ½ tsp vanilla extract

- ½ cup maple (sugar-free) syrup

Directions:

6. Preheat the waffle iron.

7. Meanwhile, in a medium bowl, mix all the ingredients until smooth.

8. Open the iron and pour in half of the mixture.

9. Close the iron and cook until crispy, 6 to 7 minutes.

10. Remove the chaffle onto a plate and set aside.

11. Make a second chaffle with the remaining batter.

12. While the chaffles cool, make the frosting.

13. Pour the almond flour in a medium saucepan and stir-fry over medium heat until golden.

14. Transfer the almond flour to a blender and top with the remaining frosting ingredients. Process until smooth.

15. 1Spread the frosting on the chaffles and
    serve afterward.

Nutrition: Calories 239 Fats 15.48g Carbs
17.42g Net Carbs 15.92g Protein 7.52g

Brie and Blackberry Chaffles

Preparation Time: 15 minutes Cooking Time: 36 minutes Servings: 4

Ingredients:

For the chaffles:

- 2 eggs, beaten

- 1 cup finely grated mozzarella cheese

For the topping:

- 1 ½ cups blackberries

- 1 lemon, 1 tsp zest and 2 tbsp juice

- 1 tbsp erythritol

- 4 slices Brie cheese

Directions:

For the chaffles:

1. Preheat the waffle iron.

2. Meanwhile, in a medium bowl, mix the eggs and mozzarella cheese.

3. Open the iron, pour in a quarter of the mixture, cover, and cook until crispy, 7

minutes.

4. Remove the chaffle onto a plate and make 3 more with the remaining batter.

5. Plate and set aside.

For the topping:

1. Preheat the oven to 350 F and line a baking sheet with parchment paper.

2. In a medium pot, add the blackberries, lemon zest, lemon juice, and erythritol. Cook until the blackberries break and the sauce thickens, 5 minutes. Turn the heat off.

3. Arrange the chaffles on the baking sheet and place two Brie cheese slices on each. Top with blackberry mixture and transfer the baking sheet to the oven.

4. Bake until the cheese melts, 2 to 3 minutes.

5. Remove from the oven, allow cooling and serve afterward.

Nutrition: Calories 576 Fats 42.22g Carbs 7.07g Net Carbs 3.67g Protein 42.35g

Cereal Chaffle Cake

Preparation Time: 5 minutes Cooking Time: 8 minutes Servings: 2

Ingredients:

- 1 egg

- 2 tablespoons almond flour

- ½ teaspoon coconut flour

- 1 tablespoon melted butter

- 1 tablespoon cream cheese

- 1 tablespoon plain cereal, crushed
  - ¼ teaspoon vanilla extract

  - ¼ teaspoon baking powder

  - 1 tablespoon sweetener

  - 1/8 teaspoon xanthan gum

Directions:

1. Plug in your waffle maker to preheat.

2. Add all the ingredients in a large bowl.

3. Mix until well blended.

4. Let the batter rest for 2 minutes before cooking.

5. Pour half of the mixture into the waffle maker.

6. Seal and cook for 4 minutes.

7. Make the next chaffle using the same steps.

Nutrition:

Calories154

Total Fat 21.2g Saturated Fat 10 g Cholesterol 113.3mg Sodium 96.9mg Potassium 453 mg Total Carbohydrate 5.9g Dietary Fiber 1.7g Protein 4.6g Total Sugars 2.7g

Chaffled Brownie Sundae

Preparation Time: 12 minutes Cooking Time: 30 minutes Servings: 4

Ingredients:

For the chaffles:

- 2 eggs, beaten

- 1 tbsp unsweetened cocoa powder

- 1 tbsp erythritol

- 1 cup finely grated mozzarella cheese

For the topping:

- 3 tbsp unsweetened chocolate, chopped

- 3 tbsp unsalted butter

- ½ cup swerve sugar

- Low-carb ice cream for topping

- 1 cup whipped cream for topping

- 3 tbsp sugar-free caramel sauce

Directions:

For the chaffles:

16. Preheat the waffle iron.

17. Meanwhile, in a medium bowl, mix all the ingredients for the chaffles.

18. Open the iron, pour in a quarter of the mixture, cover, and cook until crispy, 7 minutes.

19. Remove the chaffle onto a plate and make 3 more with the remaining batter.

20. Plate and set aside.

For the topping:

Meanwhile, melt the chocolate and butter in a medium saucepan with

occasional stirring, 2 minutes.

To Servings:

1. Divide the chaffles into wedges and top with the ice cream, whipped cream, and swirl the chocolate sauce and caramel sauce on top.

2. Serve immediately.

Nutrition: Calories 165 Fats 11.39g Carbs 3.81g Net Carbs 2.91g Protein 12.79g

Ham, Cheese & Tomato Chaffle Sandwich

Preparation Time: 5 minutes Cooking Time: 10 minutes Servings: 2

Ingredients:

- 1 teaspoon olive oil

- 2 slices ham

- 4 basic chaffles

- 1 tablespoon mayonnaise

- 2 slices Provolone cheese

- 1 tomato, sliced

Directions:

1. Add the olive oil to a pan over medium heat.

2. Cook the ham for 1 minute per side.

3. Spread the chaffles with mayonnaise.

4. Top with the ham, cheese and tomatoes.

5. Top with another chaffle to make a sandwich.

Nutrition:

Calories 198

Total Fat 14.7g Saturated Fat 6.3g Cholesterol 37mg Sodium 664mg Total Carbohydrate 4.6g Dietary Fiber 0.7g Total Sugars 1.5g Protein 12.2g Potassium 193mg

Ranch Chaffle

Preparation Time: 5 minutes Cooking Time: 8 minutes Servings: 2

Ingredients:

- 1 egg

- ¼ cup chicken cubes, cooked

- 1 slice bacon, cooked and chopped

- ¼ cup cheddar cheese, shredded

- 1 teaspoon ranch dressing powder

Directions:

1. Preheat your waffle maker.
2. In a bowl, mix all the ingredients.

3. Add half of the mixture to your waffle maker.

4. Cover and cook for 4 minutes.

5. Make the second chaffle using the same steps.

Nutrition: Calories 200 Total Fat 14 g Saturated Fat 6 g Cholesterol 129 mg Sodium 463 mg Potassium 130 mg Total Carbohydrate 2 g Dietary Fiber 1 g Protein 16 g Total Sugars 1 g

Cream Cheese Chaffle

Preparation Time: 5 minutes Cooking
Time: 8 minutes Servings: 2

Ingredients:

- 1 egg, beaten

- 1 oz. cream cheese

- ½ teaspoon vanilla

- 4 teaspoons sweetener

- ¼ teaspoon baking powder

- Cream cheese

Directions:

1. Preheat your waffle maker.

2. Add all the ingredients in a bowl.

3. Mix well.

4. Pour half of the batter into the waffle maker.

5. Seal the device.

6. Cook for 4 minutes.

7. Remove the chaffle from the waffle maker.

8. Make the second one using the same steps.

9. Spread remaining cream cheese on top before serving.

Nutrition: Calories 169 Total Fat 14.3g Saturated Fat 7.6g Cholesterol 195mg Sodium 147mg Potassium 222mg Total Carbohydrate 4g Dietary Fiber 4g Protein 7.7g Total Sugars 0.7g

Barbecue Chaffle

Preparation Time: 5 minutes

Cooking Time: 8 minutes Servings: 2

Ingredients:

- 1 egg, beaten

- ½ cup cheddar cheese, shredded

- ½ teaspoon barbecue sauce

- ¼ teaspoon baking powder

Directions:

1. Plug in your waffle maker to preheat.

2. Mix all the ingredients in a bowl.

3. Pour half of the mixture to your waffle maker.

4. Cover and cook for 4 minutes.

5. Repeat the same steps for the next barbecue chaffle.

Nutrition: Calories 295 Total Fat 23 g Saturated Fat 13 g Cholesterol 223 mg Sodium 414 mg Potassium 179 mg Total Carbohydrate 2 g Dietary Fiber 1 g Protein 20 g Total Sugars 1 g

Creamy Chicken Chaffle Sandwich

Preparation Time: 5 minutes Cooking Time: 10 minutes Servings: 2

Ingredients:

- Cooking spray

- 1 cup chicken breast fillet, cubed

- Salt and pepper to taste

- ¼ cup all-purpose cream

- 4 garlic chaffles

  - Parsley, chopped

Directions:

1. Spray your pan with oil.

2. Put it over medium heat.

3. Add the chicken fillet cubes.

4. Season with salt and pepper.

5. Reduce heat and add the cream.

6. Spread chicken mixture on top of the chaffle.

7. Garnish with parsley and top with another chaffle.

Nutrition: Calories 273 Total Fat 38.4g Saturated Fat 4.1g Cholesterol 62mg Sodium 373mg Total Carbohydrate 22.5g Dietary Fiber 1.1g Total Sugars 3.2g Protein 17.5g Potassium 177mg

Turkey Chaffle Burger

Preparation Time: 10 minutes Cooking Time: 10 minutes Servings: 2

Ingredients:

- 2 cups ground turkey

- Salt and pepper to taste

- 1 tablespoon olive oil

- 4 garlic chaffles

- 1 cup Romaine lettuce, chopped

- 1 tomato, sliced

- Mayonnaise

- Ketchup

Directions:

1. Combine ground turkey, salt and pepper. Form 2 thick burger patties.

2. Add the olive oil to a pan over medium heat.

3. Cook the turkey burger until fully cooked on both sides.

4. Spread mayo on the chaffle.

5. Top with the turkey burger, lettuce and tomato.

6. Squirt ketchup on top before topping with another chaffle.

Nutrition: Calories 555 Total Fat 21.5g Saturated Fat 3.5g Cholesterol 117mg Sodium 654mg Total Carbohydrate 4.1g Dietary Fiber 2.5g Protein 31.7g Total Sugars 1g

Bruschetta Chaffle

Preparation Time: 5 minutes Cooking
Time: 5 minutes Servings: 2

Ingredients:

- 2 basic chaffles

- 2 tablespoons sugar-free marinara
  sauce

- 2 tablespoons mozzarella, shredded

- 1 tablespoon olives, sliced

- 1 tomato sliced

- 1 tablespoon keto friendly pesto
  sauce

- Basil leaves

Directions:

1. Spread marinara sauce on each
   chaffle.

2. Spoon pesto and spread on top of the
   marinara sauce.

3. Top with the tomato, olives and mozzarella.

4. Bake in the oven for 3 minutes or until the cheese has melted.

5. Garnish with basil.

6. Serve and enjoy.

Nutrition: Calories 182 Total Fat 11g Saturated Fat 6.1g Cholesterol 30mg Sodium 508mg Potassium 1mg Total Carbohydrate 3.1g Dietary Fiber 1.1g Protein 16.8g Total Sugars 1g

Asian Cauliflower Chaffles

Preparation Time: 20 minutes Cooking Time: 28 minutes Servings: 4

Ingredients:

For the chaffles:

- 1 cup cauliflower rice, steamed

- 1 large egg, beaten

- Salt and freshly ground black pepper to taste

- 1 cup finely grated Parmesan cheese

- 1 tsp sesame seeds

- ¼ cup chopped fresh scallions

For the dipping sauce:

- 3 tbsp coconut aminos

- 1 ½ tbsp plain vinegar

- 1 tsp fresh ginger puree

- 1 tsp fresh garlic paste

- 3 tbsp sesame oil

- 1 tsp fish sauce

- 1 tsp red chili flakes

Directions:

1. Preheat the waffle iron.

2. In a medium bowl, mix the cauliflower rice, egg, salt, black pepper, and Parmesan cheese.

3. Open the iron and add a quarter of the mixture. Close and cook until crispy, 7 minutes.

4. Transfer the chaffle to a plate and make 3 more chaffles in the same manner.

5. Meanwhile, make the dipping sauce.

6. In a medium bowl, mix all the ingredients for the dipping sauce.

7. Plate the chaffles, garnish with the sesame seeds and scallions and serve with the dipping sauce.

Nutrition: Calories 231 Fats 18.88g Carbs 6.32g Net Carbs 5.42g Protein 9.66g

Hot Dog Chaffles

Preparation Time: 15 minutes Cooking Time: 14 minutes Servings: 2

Ingredients:

- 1 egg, beaten

- 1 cup finely grated cheddar cheese

- 2 hot dog sausages, cooked

- Mustard dressing for topping

- 8 pickle slices

Directions:

1. Preheat the waffle iron.

2. In a medium bowl, mix the egg and cheddar cheese.

3. Open the iron and add half of the mixture. Close and cook until crispy, 7 minutes.

4. Transfer the chaffle to a plate and make a second chaffle in the same manner.

5. To serve, top each chaffle with a sausage, swirl the mustard dressing on

top, and then divide the pickle slices on top.

6. Enjoy!

Nutrition: Calories 231 Fats 18.29g Carbs 2.8g Net Carbs 2.6g Protein 13.39g

Savory Beef Chaffle

Preparation Time: 10 minutes

Cooking Time: 15 minutes Servings: 2

Ingredients:

- 1 teaspoon olive oil

- 2 cups ground beef

- Garlic salt to taste

- 1 red bell pepper, sliced into strips

- 1 green bell pepper, sliced into strips

- 1 onion, minced

- 1 bay leaf

- 2 garlic chaffles

- Butter

Directions:

1. Put your pan over medium heat.

2. Add the olive oil and cook ground beef until brown.

3. Season with garlic salt and add bay leaf.

4. Drain the fat, transfer to a plate and set aside.

5. Discard the bay leaf.

6. In the same pan, cook the onion and bell peppers for 2 minutes.

7. Put the beef back to the pan.

8. Heat for 1 minute.

9. Spread butter on top of the chaffle.

10. 1Add the ground beef and veggies.

11. 1Roll or fold the chaffle.

Nutrition: Calories 220 Total Fat 17.8g Saturated Fat 8g Cholesterol 76mg Sodium 60mg Total Carbohydrate 3g Dietary Fiber 2g Total Sugars 5.4g Protein 27.1g Potassium 537mg

Turnip Hash Brown Chaffles

Preparation Time: 10 minutes Cooking Time: 42 minutes Servings: 6

Ingredients:

- 1 large turnip, peeled and shredded

- ½ medium white onion, minced

- 2 garlic cloves, pressed

- 1 cup finely grated Gouda cheese
- 2 eggs, beaten

- Salt and freshly ground black pepper to taste

Directions:

1. Pour the turnips in a medium safe microwave bowl, sprinkle with 1 tbsp of water, and steam in the microwave until softened, 1 to 2 minutes.

2. Remove the bowl and mix in the remaining ingredients except for a quarter cup of the Gouda cheese.

3. Preheat the waffle iron.

4. Once heated, open and sprinkle some of the reserved cheese in the iron and top with 3 tablespoons of the mixture. Close the waffle iron and cook until crispy, 5 minutes.

5. Open the lid, flip the chaffle and cook further for 2 more minutes.

6. Remove the chaffle onto a plate and set aside.

7. Make five more chaffles with the remaining batter in the same proportion.

8. Allow cooling and serve afterward.

Nutrition: Calories 230; Fats 15.85g; Carbs 5.01g; Net Carbs 3.51g; Protein 16.57g

Savory Gruyere and Chives Chaffles

Preparation Time: 15 minutes Cooking Time: 14 minutes Servings: 2

Ingredients:

- 2 eggs, beaten

- 1 cup finely grated Gruyere cheese

- 2 tbsp finely grated cheddar cheese

- 1/8 tsp freshly ground black pepper

- 3 tbsp minced fresh chives + more for garnishing

- 2 sunshine fried eggs for topping

Directions:

1. Preheat the waffle iron.

2. In a medium bowl, mix the eggs, cheeses, black pepper, and chives.

3. Open the iron and pour in half of the mixture.

4. Close the iron and cook until brown and

crispy, 7 minutes.

5. Remove the chaffle onto a plate and set aside.

6. Make another chaffle using the remaining mixture.

7. Top each chaffle with one fried egg each, garnish with the chives and serve.

Nutrition: Calories 712 Fats 41.32g Carbs 3.88g Net Carbs 3.78g Protein 23.75g

Maple Chaffle

Preparation Time: 15 minutes Servings: 2

Ingredients:

- 1 egg, lightly beaten

- 2 egg whites

- 1/2 tsp maple extract

- 2 tsp Swerve

- 1/2 tsp baking powder, gluten-free

- 2 tbsp almond milk

- 2 tbsp coconut flour

Directions:

1. Preheat your waffle maker.

2. In a bowl, whip egg whites until stiff peaks form.

3. Stir in maple extract, Swerve, baking powder, almond milk, coconut flour, and egg.

4. Spray waffle maker with cooking spray.

5. Pour half batter in the hot waffle maker and cook for 3-5 minutes or until golden brown. Repeat with the remaining batter.

6. Serve and enjoy.

Nutrition: Calories 122 Fat 6.6 g Carbohydrates 9 g Sugar 1 g Protein 7.7 g Cholesterol 82 mg

Keto Chocolate Fudge Chaffle

Preparation Time: 10 minutes Cooking Time: 14 minutes Servings: 2

Ingredients:

- 1 egg, beaten

- ¼ cup finely grated Gruyere cheese

- 2 tbsp unsweetened cocoa powder

- ¼ tsp baking powder
- ¼ tsp vanilla extract

- 2 tbsp erythritol

- 1 tsp almond flour

- 1 tsp heavy whipping cream

- A pinch of salt

Directions:

1. Preheat the waffle iron.

2. Add all the ingredients to a medium bowl and mix well.

3. Open the iron and add half of the mixture. Close and cook until golden brown and crispy, 7 minutes.

4. Remove the chaffle onto a plate and make another with the remaining batter.

5. Cut each chaffle into wedges and serve after.

Nutrition: Calories 173 Fats 13.08g Carbs 3.98g Net Carbs 2.28g Protein 12.27g

Blue Cheese Chaffle Bites

Preparation Time: 10 minutes Cooking Time: 14 minutes Servings: 2

Ingredients:

- 1 egg, beaten
- ½ cup finely grated Parmesan cheese
- ¼ cup crumbled blue cheese
- 1 tsp erythritol

Directions:

1. Preheat the waffle iron.
2. Mix all the ingredients in a bowl.
3. Open the iron and add half of the mixture. Close and cook until crispy, 7 minutes.
4. Remove the chaffle onto a plate and make another with the remaining mixture.
5. Cut each chaffle into wedges and serve afterward.

Nutrition: **Calories 196 Fats 13.91g Carbs 4.03g Net Carbs 4.03g Protein 13.48g**

Breakfast Spinach Ricotta Chaffles

Preparation Time: 10 minutes Cooking Time: 28 minutes Servings: 4

Ingredients:

- 4 oz frozen spinach, thawed, squeezed dry

- 1 cup ricotta cheese

- 2 eggs, beaten

- ½ tsp garlic powder

- ¼ cup finely grated Pecorino Romano cheese

- ½ cup finely grated mozzarella cheese

- Salt and freshly ground black pepper to taste

Directions:

1. Preheat the waffle iron.

2. In a medium bowl, mix all the ingredients.

3. Open the iron, lightly grease with cooking spray and spoon in a quarter of the mixture.

4. Close the iron and cook until brown and crispy, 7 minutes.

5. Remove the chaffle onto a plate and set aside.

6. Make three more chaffles with the remaining mixture.

7. Allow cooling and serve afterward.

Nutrition: Calories 188 Fats 13.15g Carbs 5.06g Net Carbs 4.06g Protein 12.79g

Scrambled Egg Stuffed Chaffles

Preparation Time: 15 minutes Cooking Time: 28 minutes Servings: 4

Ingredients:

For the chaffles:

- 1 cup finely grated cheddar cheese

  - 2 eggs, beaten

  For the egg stuffing:

  - 1 tbsp olive oil

- 4 large eggs

- 1 small green bell pepper, deseeded and chopped

- 1 small red bell pepper, deseeded and chopped

- Salt and freshly ground black pepper to taste

  - 2 tbsp grated Parmesan cheese

Directions:

For the chaffles:

1. Preheat the waffle iron.

2. In a medium bowl, mix the cheddar cheese and egg.

3. Open the iron, pour in a quarter of the mixture, close, and cook until crispy, 6 to 7 minutes.

4. Plate and make three more chaffles using the remaining mixture.

For the egg stuffing:

1. Meanwhile, heat the olive oil in a medium skillet over medium heat on a stovetop.

2. In a medium bowl, beat the eggs with the bell peppers, salt, black pepper, and Parmesan cheese.

3. Pour the mixture into the skillet and scramble until set to your likeness, 2 minutes.

4. Between two chaffles, spoon half of the scrambled eggs and repeat with the second set of chaffles.

5. Serve afterward.

Nutrition: Calories 387 Fats 22.52g Carbs 18.12g Net Carbs 17.52g Protein 27.76g

Lemon and Paprika Chaffles

Preparation Time: 10 minutes Cooking Time: 28 minutes Servings: 4

Ingredients:

- 1 egg, beaten

- 1 oz cream cheese, softened

- 1/3 cup finely grated mozzarella cheese

- 1 tbsp almond flour

- 1 tsp butter, melted

- 1 tsp maple (sugar-free) syrup

- ½ tsp sweet paprika

- ½ tsp lemon extract

Directions:

1. Preheat the waffle iron.

2. Mix all the ingredients in a medium bowl

3. Open the iron and pour in a quarter of the mixture. Close and cook until crispy, 7 minutes.

4. Remove the chaffle onto a plate and make 3 more with the remaining mixture.

5. Cut each chaffle into wedges, plate, allow cooling and serve.

Nutrition: Calories 48 Fats 4.22g Carbs 0.6g Net Carbs 0.5g Protein 2g

Mixed Berry- Vanilla Chaffles

Preparation Time: 10 minutes Cooking Time: 28 minutes Servings: 4

Ingredients:

- 1 egg, beaten

- ½ cup finely grated mozzarella cheese

- 1 tbsp cream cheese, softened

- 1 tbsp sugar-free maple syrup

- 2 strawberries, sliced
- 2 raspberries, slices

- ¼ tsp blackberry extract

- ¼ tsp vanilla extract

- ½ cup plain yogurt for serving

Directions:

1. Preheat the waffle iron.

2. In a medium bowl, mix all the ingredients except the yogurt.

3. Open the iron, lightly grease with cooking spray and pour in a quarter of the mixture.

4. Close the iron and cook until golden brown and crispy, 7 minutes.

5. Remove the chaffle onto a plate and set aside.

6. Make three more chaffles with the remaining mixture.

7. To Servings: top with the yogurt and enjoy.

Nutrition: Calories 78 Fats 5.29g Carbs 3.02g Net Carbs 2.72g Protein 4.32g

Chaffles with Vanilla Sauce

Serving: 6-8 chaffles (6-1/2 inches).

Preparation Time: 15 minutes Cooking Time: 30 minutes

Ingredients

- 1-2/3 cups all-purpose flour

- 4 teaspoons baking powder

- 1/2 teaspoon salt

- 2 eggs, separated

- 3-2/3 cups milk, divided

- 6 tablespoons canola oil

- 1/2 cup sugar

- 1 teaspoon vanilla extract

- 1/2 cup mozzarella cheese, shredded

- Fresh strawberries

Direction

1. In a bowl, combine flour, baking powder and salt. In another bowl, beat egg yolks lightly. Add 1-2/3 cups milk and oil; stir into dry

   ingredients just until moistened. Set aside 1/4 cup batter in a small bowl. Beat egg whites until stiff peaks form; fold into remaining batter. Add mozzarella cheese and stir well.

2. Bake in a preheated waffle iron according to manufacturer's directions until golden brown. In a saucepan, heat sugar and remaining milk until scalded. Stir a small amount into reserved batter; return all to pan. Bring to a boil; boil for 5- 7 minutes or until thickened. Remove from the heat; add vanilla and mix well (sauce will thicken upon standing). Serve over chaffles. Top with berries.

Nutrition: Calories: 429 calories Total Fat: 21g Cholesterol: 91mg Sodium: 558mg Total Carbohydrate: 50g Protein: 11g Fiber: 1g

Pecan Pumpkin Chaffle

Preparation Time: 15 minutes Servings: 2

Ingredients:

- 1 egg

- 2 tbsp pecans, toasted and chopped

- 2 tbsp almond flour

- 1 tsp erythritol

- 1/4 tsp pumpkin pie spice

- 1 tbsp pumpkin puree

- 1/2 cup mozzarella cheese, grated

Directions:

1. Preheat your waffle maker.
2. Beat egg in a small bowl.
3. Add remaining ingredients and mix well.
4. Spray waffle maker with cooking spray.
5. Pour half batter in the hot waffle maker and cook for 5 minutes or until golden brown. Repeat with the remaining batter.
6. Serve and enjoy.

Nutrition: Calories 121 Fat 9.7 g
Carbohydrates 5.7 g Sugar 3.3 g
Protein 6.7 g Cholesterol 86 mg

Cinnamon Sugar Cupcakes

- 1.5 cups Almond Flour
- 1.5 tsp Baking Powder
- ¼ tsp Salt
- ½ tsp Cinnamon
- ½ cup Erythritol
- 1/3 cup Milk
- 2 large Whole Eggs
- 1 stick Butter, softened
- 2 tsp Lemon Zest

Preparation Time: 10 minutes

Cooking Time: 25 min   Servings:6

Nutritional Values:

- Fat: 29 g.
- Protein: 8 g.
- Carbs: 7 g.

Ingredients:

Directions:

1. Preheat oven to 350F.

2. Whisk together almond flour, baking powder, cinnamon, and salt in a bowl.

3. Beat eggs, butter, and erythritol in a separate bowl. Gradually stir in the milk.

4. Stir the wet mixture into the dry ingredients.

5. Coat a 6-hole muffin pan with non-stick spray.

6. Divide the batter into the pan and bake for 25 minutes.

Coco-Blueberry Cupcakes

Preparation Time: 10 minutes

Cooking Time: 25 min Servings:6

Nutritional Values:

- Fat: 30 g.
- Protein: 6 g.
- Carbs: 7 g.

Ingredients:

- 1 cup Almond Flour
- 1/2 cup Coconut Flour
- 1 tbsp Flax Meal
- 1 tsp Baking Powder
- ¼ tsp Salt
- ½ cup Erythritol
- 1/3 cup Milk
- 2 large Whole Eggs
- ½ cup Frozen Blueberries
- ½ cup Coconut Oil

Directions:

1. Preheat oven to 350F.

2. Whisk together almond flour, coconut flour, baking pow-der, and salt in a bowl.

3. Beat eggs, coconut oil, and erythritol in a separate bowl. Gradually stir in the milk.

4. Stir the wet mixture into the dry ingredients.

5. Fold in the blueberries.

6. Coat a 6-hole muffin pan with non-stick spray.

7. Divide the batter into the pan and bake for 25 minutes.

Choco-Hazelnut Cupcakes

Preparation Time: 10 minutes

Cooking Time: 25 min Servings:6

Nutritional Values:

- Fat: 29 g.
- Protein: 9 g.
- Carbs: 9 g.
- 1.25 cup Almond Flour
- ¼ cup Unsweetened Cocoa Powder
- 1.5 tsp Baking Powder
- ¼ tsp Salt
- ½ cup Erythritol
- 1/3 cup Milk
- 2 large Whole Eggs
- 1 tsp Vanilla Extract
- 1/3 cup Hazelnut Butter
- ½ cup Sugar-Free Chocolate Chips
- ½ cup Hazelnuts, chopped

Directions:

1. Preheat oven to 350F.

2. Whisk together almond flour, cocoa powder, baking powder, and salt in a bowl.

3. Beat eggs, hazelnut butter, vanilla, and erythritol in a separate bowl. Gradually stir in the milk.

4. Stir the wet mixture into the dry ingredients.

5. Fold in the chocolate chips and hazelnuts.

6. Coat a 6-hole muffin pan with non-stick spray.

7. Divide the batter into the pan and bake for 25 minutes.

Strawberry Cream Cheese Cupcakes

Ingredients:

- 1 cup Almond Flour
- 1 tsp Baking Powder
- ¼ tsp Salt
- ½ cup Erythritol
- 1/3 cup Milk
- 2 large Whole Eggs
- 1/3 cup Cream Cheese, softened
- 1 cup Frozen Strawberries, diced

Preparation Time: 10 minutes Cooking Time: 25 min

Servings:6

Nutritional Values:

- Fat: 14 g.
- Protein: 7 g.
- Carbs: 9 g.

Directions:

2. Preheat oven to 350F.

3. Whisk together almond flour, baking powder, and salt in a bowl.

4. Beat eggs, erythritol, and cream cheese in a separate bowl. Gradually stir in the milk.

5. Stir the wet mixture into the dry ingredients.

6. Fold in the strawberries.

7. Coat a 6-hole muffin pan with non-stick spray.

8. Divide the batter into the pan and bake for 25 minutes.

Cheddar and Spinach Cupcakes

Preparation Time: 10 minutes Cooking Time: 25 min

Servings:6

Nutritional Values:

Fat: 17 g.
Protein: 9 g.
Carbs: 5 g.

Ingredients:

- 1 cup Almond Flour
- 1 tsp Baking Powder
- ¼ tsp Salt
- ½ cup Erythritol
- 1/3 cup Milk
- 2 large Whole Eggs
- 1/3 cup Cream Cheese, softened
- ½ cup Cheddar, shredded
- 1/3 cup Frozen Spinach, thawed and chopped

Directions:

1. Preheat oven to 350F.

2. Whisk together almond flour, baking powder, and salt in a bowl.

3. Beat eggs, cream cheese, and erythritol in a separate bowl. Gradually stir in the milk.

4. Stir the wet mixture into the dry ingredients.

5. Fold in the cheddar and spinach.

6. Coat a 6-hole muffin pan with non-stick spray.

7. Divide the batter into the pan and bake for 25 minutes.

Mango-Cayenne Cupcakes

Preparation Time: 10 minutes Cooking Time: 25 min

Servings:6

Nutritional Values:

Fat: 25 g.

Protein: 8 g.

Carbs: 7 g.

Ingredients:

- 1 cup Almond Flour
- 1/2 cup Coconut Flour
- 1 tbsp Flax Meal
- ½ tsp Cayenne
- 1 tsp Baking Powder
- ¼ tsp Salt
- ½ cup Erythritol
- 1/3 cup Milk
- 2 large Whole Eggs
- ½ cup Sugar-Free Mango Jelly
- ½ cup Butter, softened

1. Preheat oven to 350F.

2. Whisk together almond flour, coconut flour, baking powder, flax meal, cayenne, and salt in a bowl.

3. Beat eggs, mango jelly, butter, and erythritol in a separate bowl. Gradually stir in the milk.

4. Stir the wet mixture into the dry ingredients.

5. Coat a 6-hole muffin pan with non-stick spray.

6. Divide the batter into the pan and bake for 25 minutes.

Lime and Vanilla Cupcakes

Preparation Time: 10

minutes Cooking Time: 25

min Servings:6

Nutritional Values:

- Fat: 29 g.
- Protein: 8 g.
- Carbs: 7 g.

Ingredients:

- 1.5 cups Almond Flour
- 1.5 tsp Baking Powder
- ¼ tsp Salt
- ½ cup Erythritol
- 1/3 cup Milk
- 2 large Whole Eggs
- 1 tsp Vanilla Extract
- 1 stick Butter, softened
- 2 tsp Lime Zest

<u>Directions:</u>

1. Preheat oven to 350F.

2. Whisk together almond flour, baking powder, and salt in a bowl.

3. Beat eggs, butter, and erythritol, and vanilla in a separate bowl. Gradually stir in the milk.

4. Stir the wet mixture into the dry ingredients.

5. Fold in the lime zest.

6. Coat a 6-hole muffin pan with non-stick spray.

7. Divide the batter into the pan and bake for 25 minutes.

Chia Chocolate Cupcakes

Ingredients:

- 1.25 cup Almond Flour¼ cup Unsweetened Cocoa Powder
- 1.5 tsp Baking Powder
- ¼ tsp Salt
- ½ cup Erythritol
- 1/3 cup Milk
- 2 large Whole Eggs
- 1 tsp Vanilla Extract
- ½ cup Butter
- ½ cup Sugar-Free Chocolate Chips
- 2 tbsp Chia Seeds
-

Directions:

1. Preheat oven to 350F.
2. Whisk together almond flour, cocoa powder, baking powder, and salt in a bowl.
3. Beat eggs, butter, vanilla, and erythritol in a separate bowl. Gradually stir in the milk.
4. Stir the wet mixture into the dry ingredients.
5. Fold in the chocolate chips and chia seeds.
6. Coat a 6-hole muffin pan with non-stick spray.
7. Divide the batter into the pan and bake for 25 minutes.

Preparation Time: 10 minutes

Cooking Time: 25 min   Servings:6

Nutritional Values:

- Fat: 23 g.
- Protein: 8 g.
- Carbs: 8 g.

Keto Cheese Bread

•

Ingredients:

- 1 cup Almond Flour
- 1 tsp Baking Powder
- ¼ tsp Salt
- 1/3 cup Milk
- 2 large Whole Eggs
- 1/3 cup Cream Cheese, softened
- ½ cup Grated Parmesan

Preparation Time: 10

minutes Cooking Time: 25

min Servings:6

Nutritional Values:

- Fat: 16 g.
- Protein: 9 g.
- Carbs: 6 g.

Directions:

1. Preheat oven to 350F.

2. Whisk together almond flour, baking powder, and salt in a bowl.

3. Beat eggs and cream cheese in a separate bowl. Gradually stir in the milk.

4. Stir the wet mixture into the dry ingredients.

5. Fold in the grated parmesan.

6. Coat a 6-hole muffin tin with non-stick spray.

7. Divide the batter into the pan and bake for 25 minutes.

Keto Mug Bread

Preparation Time: 2

min Cooking Time: 2

min Servings:1

Nutritional Values:

- Fat: 37 g.
- Protein: 15 g.
- Carbs: 8 g.

Ingredients:

- 1/3 cup Almond Flour
- ½ tsp Baking Powder
    - ¼ tsp Salt
    - 1 Whole Egg
    - 1 tbsp Melted Butter

Directions:

1. Mix all ingredients in a microwave-safe mug.
2. Microwave for 90 seconds.
3. Cool for 2 minutes.

Keto Ciabatta

- 1 cup Almond Flour

Preparation Time: 1 hour

Cooking Time: 30 minutes   Servings:8

Nutritional Values:

- Fat: 11 g.
- Protein: 3 g.
- Carbs: 4 g.
- ¼ cup Psyllium Husk Powder
- ½ tsp Salt
- 1 tsp Baking Powder
- 3 tbsp Olive Oil
- 1 tsp Maple Syrup
- 1 tbsp Active Dry Yeast
- 1 cup Warm Water
- 1 tbsp Chopped Rosemary

Directions:

1. In a bowl, stir together warm water, maple syrup, and yeast. Leave for 10 minutes.

2. In a separate bowl, whisk together almond flour, psyllium husk powder, salt, chopped rosemary, and baking powder.

3. Stir in the olive oil and yeast mixture into the dry ingredients until a smooth dough is formed.

4. Knead the dough until smooth.

5. Divide the dough into 2 and shape into buns.

6. Set both buns on a baking sheet lined with parchment. Leave to rise for an hour.

7. Bake for 30 minutes at 380F.

1.

Chocolate Muffins

Serving: 10 muffins

Serving: 10 muffins Nutritional Values: Calories: 168.8,

Total Fat: 13.2 g, Saturated Fat: 1.9 g, Carbs: 19.6 g,

Sugars: 0.7 g,

Protein: 6.1 g

- Ingredients:
- 2 tsp Cream of Tartar
- 1/2 cup Erythritol
- 1 tsp Cinnamon
- Coconut Oil, for greasing

Wet ingredients:

- 2 oz medium Avocados, peeled and deseeded
- 4 Eggs
- 15-20 drops Stevia Drops
- 2 Tbsp Coconut Milk

Dry ingredients:

- 1 cup Almond Flour

- 1/3 cup Coconut Flour

- 1/2 cup Cocoa Powder

- 1 tsp Baking Soda

Directions:

1. Preheat your oven to 350F / 175C. Grease muffin cups with coconut oil and line your muffin tin.
2. Add the avocados to your food processor and pulse until smooth. Add the wet ingredients, pulse to combine until well incorporated.
3. Combine the dry ingredients and add to the food process and pulse to combine and pour the batter into your muffin tin.
4. Bake in the preheated oven for about 20-25 minutes.
5. Once crispy and baked, remove from the oven and leave to cool before serving.

Keto Blender Buns

Preparation Time: 5

minutes Cooking Time: 25

min Servings:6

Nutritional Values:

- Fat: 18 g.
- Protein: 8 g.
- Carbs: 2 g.

Ingredients:

- 4 Whole Eggs
- ¼ cup Melted Butter
- ½ tsp Salt
- ½ cup Almond Flour
- 1 tsp Italian Spice Mix

Directions:

1. Preheat oven to 425F.

2. Pulse all ingredients in a blender.

3. Divide batter into a 6-hole muffin tin.

4. Bake for 25 minutes.

Crackers with Flax Seeds

Ingredients:

- 2 tbsp flax seeds
- 1/3 cup milk
- 2 tbsp coconut oil
- 1 cup coconut flour
- ½ tsp baking powder
- 1 tsp erythritol

Prep time: 20 minutes

Nutritional Values:

- Cooking time: 20 minutes
- Servings: 10
- Calories 104
- Total carbs 10.8 g
- Protein 3 g
- Total fat 5.9 g

Directions:

1. Combine flour with baking powder, erythritol and flax seeds.

2. Gradually add milk and oil and knead the dough.

3. Wrap the dough in plastic wrap and put in the fridge for 15 minutes.

4. Divide the dough into 2 parts and roll it out with a rolling pin about 0.1 inch thick.

5. Cut out triangles.

6. Line a baking sheet with parchment paper and place the crackers on it.

7. Bake at 390°F for 20 minutes.

Rye Crackers

Ingredients:

- 1 cup rye flour
- 2/3 cup bran
- 2 tsp baking powder
- 3 tbsp vegetable oil
- 1 tsp liquid malt extract
- 1 tsp apple vinegar
- 1 cup water
- Salt to taste

Prep time: 10 minutes

- Cooking time: 15 minutes
- Servings: 10

Nutritional Values:

- Calories 80
- Total carbs 10.4 g
- Protein 1.1 g
- Total fat 4.3 g

Directions:

1. Combine flour with bran, baking powder and salt.
2. Pour in oil, vinegar and malt extract. Mix well.
3. Knead the dough, gradually adding the water.
4. Divide the dough into 2 parts and roll it out with a rolling pin about 0.1 inch thick.
5. Cut out (using a knife or cookie cutter) the crackers of square or rectangle shape.
6. Line a baking sheet with parchment paper and place the crackers on it
7. Bake at 390°F for 12–15 minutes.

Lightning Source UK Ltd.
Milton Keynes UK
UKHW020652080221
378420UK00012B/885

9 781914 203411